QUOTES   INSPIRATION
AFFIRMATIONS   WISDOM

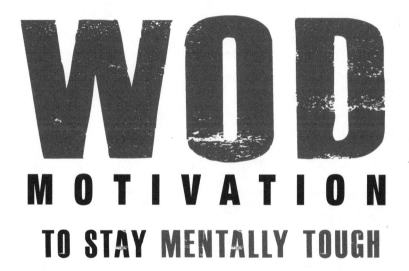

WOD

MOTIVATION
TO STAY MENTALLY TOUGH

ELEANOR BROWN, *CrossFit Journal* contributor
and *New York Times* bestselling author

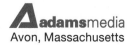

Avon, Massachusetts

Published by
Adams Media, a division of F+W Media, Inc.
57 Littlefield Street, Avon, MA 02322. U.S.A.
www.adamsmedia.com

ISBN 10: 1-4405-7061-2
ISBN 13: 978-1-4405-7061-2
eISBN 10: 1-4405-7062-0
eISBN 13: 978-1-4405-7062-9

Printed in the United States of America.

10 9 8 7 6 5 4 3 2 1

This book is not authorized, approved, licensed, or endorsed by CrossFit, Inc., which
has popularized the expression "workout of the day" and its acronym WOD. CrossFit is a
registered trademark of CrossFit, Inc.

Many of the designations used by manufacturers and sellers to distinguish their product are
claimed as trademarks. Where those designations appear in this book and F+W Media was
aware of a trademark claim, the designations have been printed with initial capital letters.

Images © 123rf.com/Samiah Binti Samin/Robertas Pezas.

This book is available at quantity discounts for bulk purchases.
For information, please call 1-800-289-0963.

INTRODUCTION

This is about more than physical strength.

In the middle of a WOD, when your legs feel like rubber and you can barely lift your arms above your waist, when you're covered in sweat and feel like you can't breathe, when the only thought you can manage to put together is that you need this to end, that is the moment when your mind must be stronger than your body.

Surviving a workout requires genuine mental toughness: the ability to talk yourself through the reps that feel impossible, to convince yourself to start the next round when you only want to rest, to finish with the same determination you had when you started. That's not easy.

But it comes with incredible payoffs. WODs change our bodies; they make us better, faster, stronger. But they also change our minds. Pushing through the challenges teaches us about ourselves—how we work, what we need, what we want. In dead lifts, we find resolve and power we never knew we had. In pull-ups, we discover a steely inner strength. Through rowing, we learn to pass through difficult waters. And when we take that knowledge forged in the box and apply it to our lives, amazing things can happen.

WOD Motivation is about that vital mental portion of your workout. There are mantras to help you make it through your toughest workouts, questions to consider when you feel your commitment flagging, and truths to make you smile and think. We're drawn to the box because of the way WODs change us on the outside, but we stay because of how they change us on the inside. May the words in this book serve as inspiration and affirmation, but mostly may they be motivation for you to get out there and kick a little ass.

On the days when the **barbell** looks like your worst enemy, make it your **best friend.**

DO FIVE.
You can always do five.

You may not ever be the best. But you can always **WORK THE HARDEST.**

When you are sure you are done, somewhere, buried deep inside you, is

ONE MORE REP.

The only thing you have to be is better than **YESTERDAY.**

They'll call you obsessed. They'll call you crazy. They'll say you've changed.

And they'll be right.

You're not the person you once were.

YOU'RE BETTER.

You must only be better, stronger, and faster than one person: **YOURSELF.**

FOCUS.
FAITH.
FORTITUDE.
FORWARD.

Tough WODs make tough people.

When everything feels complex, make it simple. Break it down, think it through, **MAKE IT HAPPEN.**

The only equipment you need is yourself.

Get your head out of your ass and get it in the **WOD**.

SHUT
UP and
lift.

Of course it's hard. It's supposed to be hard. If you wanted easy, you wouldn't be here.

When you feel your body giving up, tell your heart to **KEEP GOING.**

You don't lift the barbell with your body. You lift it with your heart, and your mind, and every ounce of courage inside you.

Do not be afraid of **failure**.

Failure is the best thing for you.

Failure is how you know you've pushed yourself hard enough.

Failure is how you know your new max.

Failure is how you determine your goal for next time.

Do not be afraid of **failure**. It is the best teacher you will ever have.

STOP
LISTENING
to people who
do not matter.

"Triumph can't be had without the struggle."

—Wilma Rudolph

Anyone who says **this is easy** ISN'T PUSHING HARD ENOUGH.

THE ONE YOU DON'T
WANT TO DO

There are days when looking at the WOD gives you a sense of anticipation and excitement. There's an exercise (or, if you're really lucky, two or three) you're really good at, or it's a WOD you haven't done in a while and you just know you'll be able to beat your previous score. There's a spring in your step and a song in your heart as you head into the box.

And then there are those other days.

Not the days when the WOD looks challenging, or when it's a metcon and you'd really rather be lifting.

No, the days when the WOD seems to have been created solely to target your weaknesses.

Run a 5k, it says, when you struggle to go more than a mile.

Burpees and hang cleans, it says, when burpees exhaust you immediately and your elbows are always too slow and too low on your cleans.

Toes to bar, it says, when you've never figured out how to get a rhythm going, making each one an exhausting grind.

These are the days when you least want to do the WOD. But these are the days when you absolutely have to do it. In fact, the less you want to do that particular workout, the more you must.

There is only one way to improve your weaknesses: practice. There is only one way to defeat your fears: face them. If you love to run and hate to row, when your coach offers you a choice between running and rowing, you must choose rowing. If you are terrified of box jumps, you must make time to work on them even when they are not part of the WOD. If snatching feels awkward and uncomfortable, you must get a PVC pipe and practice the move again and again and again until it feels so natural you don't even have to think about it.

The days where the WOD seems designed for you are like a gift. Those are the days that make you feel like a champion, that let you show off and spend the rest of the day mentally pumping your fist in the air whenever you think of how amazing you are. But they're also there to carry you through the days when the WOD seems like it's made to punish you. On those days, there may be no spring in your step, no song in your heart, no joy in the movements. But those are the days you get better. Those are the days that make the difference. Those are the most important days of all.

There is no such day as someday.

DON'T GIVE UP.

You are going to be amazing.

This is a process, not a miracle.

Be proud of your ACCOMPLISHMENTS, but never let them be enough.

What you did yesterday

is nothing in comparison to what you will do **today**.

GO FORTH AND BE AWESOME.

Every **FAILURE** is a step on the road to **SUCCESS.**

"And though she be but little, she is fierce."

—William Shakespeare,
A Midsummer Night's Dream

POSITIVE
results come from
POSITIVE
thoughts.

What is wrong with starting at the bottom? Everything you do there lifts you one step higher.

You don't have to lift the heaviest weight.
Just lift.

You don't have to run the fastest.
Just run.

You don't have to jump the highest.
Just jump.

You don't have to finish first.
Just finish.

You don't have to be the best.
Just be your best.

3, 2, 1, GO.

There is no space in my mind for anything but **EXCELLENCE.**

YOU FEEL WEAK.

YOU'RE TIRED.

YOU WANT TO GIVE UP.

DON'T.

WHAT DO WE TRAIN FOR?

We train to run across the street before the light changes.

We train to carry our children up the stairs to bed.

We train to catch our elderly parents before they fall.

We train to carry our groceries in from the car.

We train to bend and lift and reach and push and pull our way through the day.

This is fitness for the things that matter.

We train for life.

When your body tells you it can't do one more rep?

DO ONE MORE REP.

This is not about how many miles you can run.

This is not about your new max dead lift.

This is not about your ten-minute AMRAP score.

This is not about ANYTHING BUT YOU and your future and all the ways you will make yourself amazing.

Powered by **IRON**, **CALLUSES**, and **SWEAT**.

If you want to be a champion, you are going to need to work your ass off. **STARTING RIGHT NOW.**

If you are trying to be like everyone else, how will you ever become **extraordinary?**

Easy is the danger zone.

Easy means you have given up.

Easy means you have accepted what everyone else has said about you.

Easy means you have decided you no longer matter.

BE HARD ON YOURSELF.

DON'T WORRY
about how long it takes.

DON'T WORRY
about how hard it feels.

DON'T WORRY
about how many times you
think you can't.

You can.

DO IT.

Make yourself

BEG

for mercy.

The workout is as hard or as easy as you make it. **You are in control.**

The **WORST DAYS** are the ones where you look at the

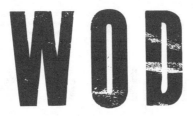

and think,
"That doesn't look so bad."

We don't do this because it's easy (it's not).

We don't do this because it's fun (it is).

We do this because it matters.

WHERE THE MAGIC HAPPENS

Everyone has that moment in a workout. That moment when you are sure it is over, that you cannot finish, you cannot go on for even another second. There are five reps, seven reps, a dozen reps left, and you are positive you don't have even one left inside you.

This is the moment that matters.

This is where the magic happens.

If you stop now, you have not failed. You have done exactly as much as you thought you could, and you have probably gotten a damn good workout in the process.

But nothing has changed.

But if you don't stop? If you keep going? If you dig deep within yourself, pushing yourself to tears, looking into the eyes of your coach who is bending down beside you, listening to the voice inside yourself and the shouts of encouragement from the athletes around you telling you that you can do this, you can make it, you've got this?

That is where the magic happens.

The reps don't matter. The weight doesn't matter. What matters is what you have found inside yourself, that you have pushed yourself further than you thought you could go.

This is not about the gym. This is not about PR's or Rx's or whether you've improved from the last time you did this WOD. This is about you and what happens in this box that you can take with you to help you push through the times in your life when you think, "I can't."

There is no magic in the weight, in lifting barbells up and putting them back down, in swinging kettlebells, in push-ups, pull-ups, Turkish get-ups, or whatever kind of special torture your coach has programmed for you.

The magic is inside you, and it only comes out when you think there is nothing there at all. Dig deep. Find the magic and make it happen.

When you feel afraid,
be brave.

When you feel empty,
be full.

When you feel weak,
be strong.

Haters
gonna hate.
Don't do their job for them.

DONE is better than FUN.

What you do when there are **three seconds left** on the clock shows **who you are.**

Your body was made to do this. You were made to run and jump and squat and swing and lift and drop and bend and roll. Your lungs want to gasp for breath; your heart wants to pound. This is completely natural, and you were born to do it. Be thankful for the miracle of your body and let it do what it was made for.

We are not here for the champions.

We are here to *make* champions.

SIGNS OF A GOOD WORKOUT:

Can't walk.

Can't sit down.

Can't breathe.

Can't think straight.

Can't wait to do it again.

Every **WOD** asks two questions: **who are you, and who do you want to be?**

You will only become

STRONGER

by using up every last ounce of strength you have.

Scaling a workout
does not make it easier.

Scaling a workout
makes you better.

It's not impossible.
YOU JUST HAVEN'T DONE IT BEFORE.

OUTSIDE THE BOX

What you do in the gym makes a difference in your life. All of this? The sweat and the iron and the rope burns and the bruises? They have changed who you are.

Fear and anxiety have a way of making us forget our strengths. So remember this: You are no longer afraid of a barbell, a pull-up rack, a sled, or a kettlebell, so why would you still be afraid of your boss, your family, a bully, a neighbor?

You make incredible things happen in the gym. But you need to carry those lessons outside the box.

When you think you can't possibly chase your dream, you must remind yourself that you can run.

When you feel afraid to speak in front of a crowd, you must remind yourself that you have lifted heavier weights than your anxiety.

When you think a step outside your comfort zone—asking for a raise, standing up to your siblings, starting your own business—is too big, remember there was once a time when you thought you couldn't do a box jump.

In every workout, you push yourself beyond what you thought you were capable of. You must allow yourself to do the same outside the box. The lessons you learn inside these four walls matter. They haven't just made you a better athlete. They have made you a different person.

The people you work out with have seen you at your best. Cast off your fear and let the rest of the world see you that way, too.

The strongest you will ever be is when you are lifting **someone else's spirits.**

We are in this together.

Cheer for me. Push me to be my best. Never let me give up. When I fall, give me a hand up. When I am scared, tell me I can do it, and I will do the same for you.

No one else is judging you. You are judging yourself.

Your body is
NOT
a garbage can.

"I am building a fire, and every day I train, I add more fuel. At just the right moment, I light the match."

—Mia Hamm

Right now you are not the best you will ever be, but you are the **BEST YOU HAVE EVER BEEN.**

Make your goals small, and celebrate every single step of the way.

Today I will put aside my expectations. Today I will accept where I am and be proud of all I have accomplished, instead of dwelling on how much further I have to go. Today I will put aside the "should" and the "should have" and focus on the "can" and the "will do." Today I will only ask myself to do the very best I can at this moment, and I will celebrate and be grateful for everything I can do.

WWYCS?

What would your coach say?

Keep
your eye
on the bar.

You could spend your time at the gym comparing your achievements to everyone else's, your body to everyone else's, sizing up times and weights and rounds. Or you could narrow your vision, focus on your own workout, and do the very best that you can do today.

One of these is a path to success and happiness. The other leads to jealousy and self-hatred.

YOU CHOOSE.

FAILURE
and **DEFEAT**
are not the same thing.

ATTITUDE Bravery. Community.

Dedication. EFFORT. FOCUS

Goals. Heart. **Intensity.**

JOY. KINDNESS Learning.

Motivation. **Nature.** OPTIMISM.

PRACTICE Quality. Respect.

Sweat. TOUGHNESS. UNITY

Vision. Wisdom. **eXpertise.**

YOUTHFULNESS. ZEAL

We cheer for the strongest, the fastest, the champions.

We cheer for the weakest, the slowest, those who never believed they could do it.

We cheer for the ones in the middle, who show up day after day and simply get it done.

We cheer for everyone with the heart to make it happen. No exceptions.

"Strength does not come from physical capacity. It comes from an indomitable will."

—Mahatma Gandhi,
"The Doctrine of the Sword"

I am grateful for my body.

I am thankful for the things it allows me to do.

I do not criticize it for the things it cannot do.

I appreciate its strengths and I accept its weaknesses.

I do not compare it to others.

I recognize its beauty.

I respect its limits.

I keep it safe and do not push it to injury.

I tend to its needs before, during, and after a workout.

I fill it with love and strength when it feels weak.

I do not take its abilities for granted.

When it feels like there's too much on your plate, get a bigger plate.

I AM FIERCE.

I AM POWERFUL.

I AM STRONG.

I AM A FORCE TO BE
RECKONED WITH.

PRIDE AND EGO

There is a difference between pride and ego.

Pride pushes you to be your best. Ego is anxiety and weakness that demands you look or perform better than anyone else.

Pride is what you feel when you celebrate a new PR. Ego is the jealousy you feel when someone else's new PR is faster or heavier than yours.

Pride drives you to finish when you are tired. Ego ignores your body's signals and pushes you past your limits into injury.

Pride is internal. Ego is external, constantly looking at the performance of others and judging yourself to be the loser every time.

This is why, when you enter a box, you are told to leave your ego at the door. Taking your ego into a WOD is dangerous, both to your body and your mind. Your ego leaves you with a disappointed heart and damaged muscles.

Egos are sticky, tricky things. You think you've left it behind, and then it sneaks up in the middle of a lift, whispering, "Look at how much heavier her bar is; what's wrong with you?" or "Form isn't so important—*time* is what matters, and look at how slow you are." When you are tired and focused on getting it done, and that voice is so much louder than the reason of your muscles and your tendons and your breath, it is so easy to fall under its spell.

It takes practice, ignoring the voice of your ego. But it's worth it in the end. Because the promises of your ego are lies. When you sacrifice form for time, there is no pride in the score. When you injure yourself because you have moved too fast or lifted too heavy, there is no pride in the pain.

And pride is what you are after. Pride is what you want—that limitless, happy feeling when you have done the very best you could, and done it right, and done it honestly. That is why you are here.

THINGS TO LOSE:

Your excuses.

Your fear.

Your weakness.

Your jealousy.

Your ego.

Your expectations.

THINGS TO KEEP:

Your ideals.

Your goals.

Your hope.

Your intensity.

Your resolve.

Your self-respect.

The good news is that the first time you do anything, no matter how you perform, you're guaranteed a PR.

You **will** wish you had kept fighting. But you **will not** wish you had surrendered.

We respect each other here. We don't diminish people's strengths, and we don't mock their weaknesses. We share our frustrations and our achievements, our victories and our failures. We are in this for ourselves, and we are in this for each other. We are in this together.

Stop looking over your shoulder and GET YOUR MIND ON YOUR OWN BAR.

This is not just a box jump. This is a leap of faith in yourself.

The true champion in the gym is not the person who can lift the most or run the fastest. The true champion is the one who looks at the workout and says, "I can't do this, but I'm doing it anyway."

RUN like someone just set your ass on FIRE.

How will you know unless you try?

In most **WOD**s,

the basic goal is just

not to die.

This is **difficult** and **painful**

and **exhausting** and **terrifying**

and **exciting** and **amazing** and

thrilling and **miraculous**, and

I LOVE EVERY SINGLE MOMENT OF IT.

Less talky, more worky.

"In the depths of winter, I finally learned that within me there lay an invincible summer."

—Albert Camus, "Return to Tipasa"

Why worry about tomorrow? There is work to be done today.

Every day is different. There are days when you will be weak and days when you will be strong. Some days the weight will feel impossible, and other days that same weight will move as though it is part of your body, as though it is meant to be.

Some days your feet and your breath will work together and you will run as though you had been born to do it. Some days every step will feel as if your legs were made of lead. Some days you will be the fastest. Some days you will finish last.

It's worth asking why—sleep and food and stress and form all matter. But sometimes it just is what it is, and then comes the hard part: letting go.

So it wasn't a PR. So you didn't reach your goal. So it was harder than last time, or harder than you thought it would be. So it wasn't better than everyone else in the box, or better than your previous time. Sometimes you can evaluate your performance and find a reason for it—you ate poorly, you slept poorly, your heart wasn't in it. Some days, there's no reason at all. You ate poorly, slept poorly, and you rocked out a PR. Or you ate well, slept well, and moved like a turtle swimming in syrup. It's a mystery.

So what?

There are days like that. There are days when things are amazing. There are days when things go horribly wrong. But they're just days. They pass, they're over, and a new one comes along. And here's the real miracle: with that new day comes a whole new opportunity. Maybe it will be the same, maybe it will be worse, maybe it will be better. But no matter which it is, you take it as it comes, you learn from it, and then, most importantly, you move on, grateful that there will be another chance, another day.

Every day is an **opportunity** to prove to yourself that you are stronger than you ever could have imagined.

There are no limits to my strength.

There is a limit to my weakness, but there are no limits to my strength.

I am not here to make my body strong. **I am here to strengthen my mind, my heart, and my spirit.** What happens to my body is a side effect.

The best way to
put a bad

WOD

behind you is
to cheer your
hardest for
someone else.

Some days the wall ball is just going to hit you in the face.

Don't just exercise.
Inspire yourself.

This community does not judge you by what you look like, what kind of car you drive, or how much money you make. What matters here are your heart and soul and the energy you bring with you every day.

STOP
THINKING
SO MUCH.

"Progress is impossible without change, and those who cannot change their minds cannot change anything."

—George Bernard Shaw

KNOW THYSELF

You know yourself by now.

You know whether looking at the workout ahead of time is going to pump you up for the challenge or make you cancel your reservation.

When you are setting up for the workout, you know whether you tend to underestimate your strength and go too easy on yourself or ignore your body's messages and end up injured. You know whether you listen to your coach and your log book and program the workout that's right for you, or whether you look at the people around you and choose your modifications based on your ego instead of your needs.

During the WOD, you know the script that runs in your mind and tells you that it's too hard or you're too weak, and you know the magic words to make that voice go away. You know what works for you—counting your breaths, ignoring the clock or staring at it, listening to the music or tuning it out. You know what gets you through.

The problem is not that you do not know what works for you. You know yourself. The problem is that you are not applying that knowledge to make yourself better. You are allowing yourself to be distracted by your ego or other people's opinions of you or other people's goals for themselves or a million other things that are irrelevant to who you are and what you need right now.

You know your strengths and you know your weaknesses. You know what you want, and you know what's stopping you. Take that knowledge and make it happen.

It takes 10,000 hours of practice to become an expert?

YOU'D BETTER GET GOING.

Like a boss.

The best thing you can do for yourself is to get out of your own way.

You are
not
finished yet.

I build **opportunities** out of obstacles.

I turn challenges into **victories**.

I create **knowledge** from failure.

I forge positive **results** from negative events.

I make **miracles** happen every day.

You don't have to finish first. You just have to finish.

Some days, **HONOR** and **VICTORY** are found in simply showing up and getting it done.

Blessed are those who lift, for they shall become strong enough to carry their problems.

Blessed are those who run, for they shall have the endurance to move through difficult times.

Blessed are those who stretch, for they shall be flexible enough to withstand the winds of change.

Blessed are those who sweat, for they shall know the value of hard work.

You will
thank yourself
tomorrow.

Neither success nor failure is permanent.

Remember

when you thought you

couldn't?

Ask yourself if what you are doing is bringing you closer to your goals.

THIS IS HOW WE **ROW**.

A rest day is not an admission of weakness. A rest day is an offering of gratitude to your body. A rest day is an opportunity for your muscles to heal and grow stronger. A rest day gives you the chance to push twice as hard the day before and the day after. A rest day is a chance to sleep, and spend time with your family, and read, and go for a walk, and to remember there is as much beauty in trees and leaves as there is in bumpers and chalk. A rest day is a gift.

You are not just building your body.

You are feeding your soul.

JUST ONE MORE.

ONE MORE REP.

ONE MORE SWING.

ONE MORE STEP.

ONE MORE PUSH.

ONE MORE PULL.

ONE MORE BREATH.

ONE MORE SQUAT.

ONE MORE STROKE.

JUST ONE MORE.

It's okay if you're **intimidated.** I'm kind of **awesome.**

" . . . the harder the conflict, the more glorious the triumph."

—Thomas Paine, *The American Crisis*

I will not be ashamed of the things I have worked so hard for.

I DON'T CARE WHAT YOU LOOK LIKE. **SHOW ME WHAT YOU CAN DO.**

"How come you never talk about your workouts?"

said no one ever.

LITTLE GOALS

Everyone loves setting big goals. One hundred unbroken double-unders. A handstand walk from one end of the box to the other. A twenty-minute 5k. Improving a benchmark WOD time by more than a minute.

We're not so good at figuring out how to get to those big goals. The bigger the goal, the more exciting it is. It is easy to see the victory parade at the end, to imagine the feeling of triumph, to envision the accolades and admiration. But the longer it takes to reach that goal, and the further those rewards seem, the easier it is to get discouraged.

So what do we do in the meantime?

We need to get better at setting little goals. These tiny steps are what take us forward toward the big goal. These smaller achievements may not be parade-worthy, but they keep us going from day to day, or from moment to moment.

There is no goal too small. In the hardest WOD, the tiniest goals can be exactly what we need to make it through. Just keep going until the next chorus of the song. Just keep going until the next lamppost. Just keep going for the next five seconds. Every one of those can feel like an achievement. Put enough of them together and the workout is done.

One hundred double-unders can seem distant and defeating. But what about five minutes of practice every day for a week? Twenty unbroken pull-ups is impossible. What about two pull-ups without a break? And then four? And then six?

And we must learn to *celebrate* those small goals. We must learn to announce the small triumphs and to applaud and reward our successes.

The big dreams may be the reason we get up in the morning, but the little goals are the ones that help us make it through the minutia of every day.

Set a small goal. Aim for it, achieve it, and then do it all over again. That is how to reach the victory parade.

"You gain strength, courage, and confidence by every experience in which you stop to look fear in the face. . . . You must do the thing you think you cannot do."

—Eleanor Roosevelt, *You Learn by Living*

You have never been more beautiful than when you are:

SWEATING.
STRAINING.
STRUGGLING.
SCREAMING.
STRETCHING.
SUFFERING.
SUCCEEDING.

Let the world fall away. Let the noise disappear. Let the only sound you hear be the rush of your blood and the beating of your heart and the beauty of your breath coming ragged and hard. Feel the grip of your hands, the cool metal, the press of your feet on the floor. This is all that matters: the moment and you in it, and what you are about to do. Ready? Set? Go.

Haven't you always wanted to be more than you are?

This is more than what we do.

THIS IS WHO WE ARE.

If you can't do *everything*, you can still do *something*.

I can go from **zero to awesome** in **four beeps of the clock.**

WHAT
is stopping you?

Just because you're a **beauty** doesn't mean you can't be a **BEAST.**

Good morning, sunshine! How about we kick a little ass today?

Modify your workouts.
Rx YOUR LIFE.

YOU ARE NOT HERE FOR THE BARS. You are not here for the kettlebells and the pull-up rig. You are not here for the chalk, or the medicine balls, or the plyo boxes, or the tires.

YOU ARE HERE FOR THE PEOPLE. You are here for the shouts of encouragement. You are here for the high-five from your coach for a job well done. You are here for the moments when you find strength you did not know you had, and you are here for the times you see someone else do the same.

YOU COME FOR THE WORKOUT, BUT YOU STAY FOR WHAT MATTERS.

Do not look at how far you have to go. *Look at how far you have come.*

"There is no living thing that is not afraid when it faces danger. The true courage is in facing danger when you are afraid."

—L. Frank Baum,
The Wonderful Wizard of Oz

Make your **last rep** as good as your **first**.

When life gets you down, pick up a bar.

CHASING THE Rx

So you want to Rx your WOD. Welcome to the club.

You get to the box, check out the WOD on the board, and after you've recovered from the initial shock, you focus on the particulars of what your coach is asking you to do.

Sometimes, you know there's no way an Rx is going to happen. The WOD calls for pull-ups, and you do banded pull-ups. The WOD calls for double-unders, and you don't have them yet. Rx just isn't in the cards for you that day.

And sometimes, it feels temptingly close. You can totally do a 125-pound dead lift. Ten times in a row? Well, you'd feel better if it were 115, but you're sure you can do it, as long as you don't focus too much on your time. Box jumps? Well, you usually do 18 inches, but if Rx is 20, you'll figure out a way. You forgot your knee socks and you may end up with a few scrapes, but it'd be worth it to see that Rx after your name on the board.

Before you make your decision, try looking at it from this perspective:

You are already Rx-ing every single workout you do.

You are doing every workout as prescribed . . . *for you*.

Maybe your prescription is not the same as the one on the board. That's okay. The Rx on the board? It's *supposed* to be hard. It's supposed to be a goal to aim for, a standard to reach. And in the meantime, you use it as a guideline, and you consult with yourself, your coach, and your log book, and you figure out your own personal Rx.

You're doing the workout as prescribed . . . *for you*.

You're doing banded or jumping pull-ups because that's *your* prescribed method right now. You're swinging a 25-pound kettlebell because that's *your* prescribed weight right now. You're jumping on a 16" box or stepping up to a 12" box because that's *your* prescribed height right now. That, my friend, is a true Rx.

If it makes you feel better, substitute your first initial for the "R" in "Rx" and put that on the board next to your score. Michael? You just Mx'd that WOD. Jennifer? Congratulations on Jx-ing the WOD!

Rx is just letters. Do what you need to get the most out of every workout.

Just for you.

You can rest when you have finished.

Every MASTER was once a BEGINNER.

COMPLAIN

AS MUCH AS YOU

WANT—JUST

GET IT DONE.

Extend the same kindness to yourself that you do to others.

THE CLOCK IS
not interested
in bargaining with you.

JUST IMAGINE: Most people go their entire lives without ever experiencing this kind of achievement, and you get to feel it **every single day**.

If you'd started

WODing

when you started

worrying, you'd be

done by now.

You can **focus** on what you *can't* do, or you can **celebrate** what you *can*.

There is no problem
a good WOD
can't cure.

This is not about punishing your body. This is about celebrating all the amazing things it can do.

Tomorrow you will smile

when you feel sore, and you will remember that today you did something you did not think you could do.

nguvu mani 힘

fuerza

kraft 力量 força

STRENGTH

δύναμη

force forza

сила 力 styrke

At what other point in your day will you get to do something just for you?

YOU ARE NOT ALONE

In the midst of a WOD, it can feel like you're all alone. Community takes a back seat when the clock beeps and the coach shouts, "Go!" Everyone focuses on themselves and what they're trying to get done.

And that's not a bad thing. People have their own goals each day: Some are trying to set PR's, some are just trying not to pass out. Whatever it is, you have to crawl inside your own mind, pay attention to your body, and do what it takes to make it through.

It's easy to think—when you're working so hard, when the sweat is pouring off you in sheets, when your breath is coming shallow and rough and your muscles are whispering to you how nice and how comfortable it would be for you to take a break, or maybe to stop altogether, it's easy to think that no one else is feeling the same way. From the outside, it seems no one else is finding this as hard as you are, no one else is struggling to keep going, no one else is gasping for breath. In fact, everyone else is making it look easy. They're swinging through their kipping pull-ups, they're rowing with long, easy strokes, they're finishing their sit-ups in unbroken sets. When you are struggling, watching someone else can be discouraging. It can make you feel like you are the only one for whom this is difficult.

Here is the truth: No matter how easy they make it look, everyone around you is struggling. Their struggles may be different than yours, but they exist. They're struggling with their form, or their cardiovascular endurance, or the voice in their head that tells them they can't do it. They're recuperating from an injury, recovering from a bad night's sleep, or trying to forget about their problems at work.

From the outside, you cannot tell what is going on in someone's workout, or their head, or their life. But one thing is certain—nothing is what it seems. The person with the perfect body you covet may be filled with insecurities and problems. The weakest and slowest member of the gym may have an inner strength worthy of envy. The only thing that is guaranteed is that everyone is working through something. You are not the only one. Don't spend your time wondering why it looks so much easier for someone else. It's not easy for them. It's not easy for anyone. You are not alone.

I'm not going to kick anyone's ass.

(But it sure is nice to know I could.)

The **WOD** has a way of trying to mess with your mind. That's its job. Your job is not to let it.

It could be worse.
It could be
THRUSTERS.

BEFORE YOU QUIT, YOU MUST ASK YOURSELF TWO QUESTIONS:

What is the **best** that could happen if I kept going?

What is the **worst** that could happen if I stopped?

Find the person at your box who inspires you and work out with them. Use their energy to keep yourself moving; to push hard and finish strong.

"Victory belongs to the most persevering."

—Napoleon Bonaparte

The bar has no pity. The bar has no compassion. The bar does not care if you have had a hard day, or if you are tired or scared. The bar will not adjust itself to suit your desires. The bar meets you on its terms. The only way to survive is to make yourself as tough as the bar.

You will never learn as much about yourself as you will during a

WOD.

I may be in last place, but at least I'm on the board.

A GOOD COACH . . .

. . . shows you the difference between your fears and your abilities.

. . . knows when you need a break and when you're just being lazy.

. . . makes you laugh when you want to scream.

. . . inspires you to challenge yourself.

. . . teaches you how to find your limits, then move beyond them.

. . . understands why you're crying, but won't let you quit.

. . . acts as your biggest fan and your toughest critic.

. . . gives you his or her time, knowledge, and energy.

. . . appears by your side when you need it most.

. . . is a gift and an inspiration.

SLOPPY FORM **does not make** TIGHT ABS.

Release your inner beast.

ALL YOU REALLY NEED TO KNOW ABOUT LIFE YOU LEARN AT THE GYM

Clean up after yourself.

Everybody shares the chalk.

If you put it down, you're going to have to pick it back up.

Nothing makes you feel better than encouraging other people.

Come early, stay late, and work your ass off in between.

Once you get going, you'll be too busy to be scared.

I love getting angry. I love the feeling of fury inside me, like a hurricane pushing me through the **WOD**. I love stomping and shouting and cursing my way through each movement. I love taking the aggression and forging strength from it, like iron in fire. My wrath makes me powerful. My rage cleanses me. My anger makes me mighty and strong.

CHEAPER
than therapy.

"My legs can keep no pace with my desires."

—William Shakespeare,
A Midsummer Night's Dream

You may have to crawl your way out of the box when it's over, but at least you're still crawling.

Just because you are not yet a **complete success** does not mean you are a **total failure**.

If it's all too much.

If you can't think.

If you can't keep track of your reps.

If you can't focus on technique.

Then just breathe.

Make breathing your only job.

All you have to do is keep air moving in and out of your body, feeding your blood, your muscles, your brain, and your heart.

That's all you have to do.

Just keep breathing.

Your **WOD** is the most important meeting you have all day, with your most important client: **yourself.**

DO NOT CANCEL.

NOTHING WILL MAKE YOU WEAKER THAN BELIEVING YOU WILL NEVER BE STRONG.

Do not compare—
COMPETE.

When it feels **HARD,** tell yourself it is **EASY.**

When have
you ever not
been able to
do one more?

Sometimes you have to go through a **PERSONAL WORST** on the way to a **PERSONAL BEST.**

BOO FLIPPING HOO.

The problem is not that your legs are not strong enough. **The problem is that your mind is not strong enough.**

BETWEEN YOU AND YOURSELF

You are the only person who knows how you feel today. You are the only person who knows how your body is doing after your other workouts this week. You are the only person who can evaluate your energy level and your pain level and the states of your body and your mind. You are the only person who can set your goals for today.

Only you will see every single movement in this WOD, and only you will know whether each one was perfectly executed. Only you will know if you shorten your range of motion, or change the weight, or add a modification halfway through. Only you will see the corners you cut or witness the extra rep you do when you have lost count.

If you quit, you will be the only person affected. If you cheat your reps or your rounds, you are only cheating yourself. If you allow your body to control your mind, only you know the effects. If you push through discomfort or stop because of pain, it is your decision alone.

Your coach will encourage you, but cannot force you. The other athletes will cheer for you, but cannot finish your workout for you. The clock will be a reminder, but you must stay focused on your own.

You are setting the standards. You are controlling your experience. You are your only competition. For better or for worse, this WOD is just between you and yourself.

Go ahead.

TELL ME I CAN'T DO THIS.

You can do anything for one minute.

Some days you kill the WOD.

Some days the WOD kills you.

How about this time you try thinking of all the reasons you can?

In this box, we are family.
So if you die during the

WOD ,

we promise to give you a
real nice funeral.

You will never **succeed** if you are constantly preparing for **failure.**

Think of all the people you are proving wrong.

The rep

that matters most
is the one you are
sure you cannot do.

NO:

Doubt

Quitting

Criticism

Whining

ONLY:

Trust

Commitment

Respect

Winning

If you make half-hearted efforts, you will get half-assed results.

Do not focus so much on being strong that you forget to be flexible.

What is flexible cannot be broken.

Even a stone can be changed with enough time, pressure, and heat.

I am a secret SUPERHERO. With an invisible cape.

Get the movement started, and the weight will do the rest.

PUSH IT. PULL IT.
LIFT IT. SLAM IT.
DROP IT. SWING IT.
HOLD IT. CARRY IT.
FLIP IT. BEND IT.
SQUAT IT. REPEAT.

BRING IT ALL IN

You must bring everything to your workout. You must bring all of your strength, your determination, and your energy, but you must also bring the bad things: the fight with your partner, your concerns about money, your frustration with your children, and your anxiety about work.

You have come to the box not to forget those problems but to solve them. The WOD will help you do that, but you must offer your problems up to the workout. You must put them on the bar with the weight. You must lay them on the pavement when you run and let yourself pass over them. You must throw them in the air with the wall ball.

There are days when your problems seem too heavy to carry. On those days you may not earn your fastest time or your best score. But on those days you don't need numbers to carry you through. On those days what you really need is to WOD your way through your problems. You need to lift the bar so you know you can lift your worries. You need to wrap your hands around the solid metal of the pull-up rig so you are reminded that things can be stable and grounded. You need to hop on the bike and pedal so your feet remind you that life moves in cycles.

If you hold back, if you do not release your problems to the workout, you will not be able to fully commit to it, and you will not reap the benefits. But if you enter with your whole heart, you have the chance to leave it all on the floor when you are finished. You can sweat out the shame and the regret and the ego. You can leave the heavy weights on the bar and walk out with high hopes and a clear head.

If you survive the WOD, you will see that you can survive your problems. But you can only do that if every part of you is here—the good and the bad.

YOU ARE NOT
THE KIND OF PERSON
WHO RETREATS
FROM A
CHALLENGE.

You will never run out of excuses.

You will only run out of time.

THERE IS POWER IN MY LEGS.

THERE IS POWER IN MY ARMS.

THERE IS POWER IN MY LUNGS.

THERE IS POWER IN MY CORE.

THERE IS POWER IN MY FEET.

THERE IS POWER IN MY HIPS.

THERE IS POWER IN MY HEART.

THERE IS POWER IN MY MIND.

W O D

like there's no
tomorrow.